Renal Diet

Booklet

Cookbook for the Newly Diagnosed with Kidney-Friendly Recipes that areTasty & Easy to Prepare.

Estelle Farmer

TABLE OF CONTENTS

INTRODUCTION

Two recent findings suggest that a high protein diet, which is often recommended as a way to lose weight and improve health, is detrimental to the kidneys of people with seemingly normal kidney function. Chronic kidney disease (CKD) is associated with a low-protein diet, which has been found in several trials to damage kidney function. According to a new study, progressive kidney disorders like kidney failure and kidney cancer can be treated with a high-protein diet, which is why nephrologists tend to prescribe it to patients in the early stages of the condition. Seeking natural strategies to reduce high blood pressure will also help protect the kidneys, according to a new report, since it is a risk factor for kidney disease.

Kidney-friendly recipes, prepared by a chef and a dietitian, are suitable for kidney feeding. There is dietary information and meals given in an easy-to-read format, and if you're like me, you can speak to me about creating a menu that works for you.

This is an area of your diet that you can keep an eye on if you have kidney disease. Even if your kidney diet restricts protein, you must consume high-quality protein during the day.

Excess protein will place a burden on the kidneys if kidney function is already compromised. To keep the kidneys running, it's essential to eat the right amount of high-quality, high-protein foods. Consult your kidney dietitian on combining the 15 right ingredients into a balanced eating regimen for your kidney diet. Remember to eat the way you want to after you've understood which foods are healthy for you on a kidney diet and which are poor. You can need to change your dietary habits if you exercise too much and eat too little, or if you inherit polycystic kidney disease, so your kidneys are not working as well as they once were.

Carbohydrates are high in potassium and phosphorus, all of which you can need to restrict based on the kidney disease level. Your dietician can recommend special supplements designed for people with kidney disease to ensure you get the right amount of vitamins and minerals. You will need a phosphorus-free calcium supplement or calcium supplements such as calcium chloride if you have chronic kidney disease.

If you use whole grains in your kidney diet, it will be enriched and provide all of the fiber you need for health benefits, as well as potentially enough protein without increasing your phosphorus intake. Diversify the diet by including low-sodium foods like whole beans, whole grains, and whole rice. If you include whole grains in a kidney diet, you can get all of the fiber you need for their health benefits, as well as adequate protein due to the increased phosphorus content, as well as diet diversification - a low sodium option. Whole beans, almonds, peas, legumes, vegetables, fruits, grains, and nuts are high-fibre, low-sodium ingredients that are used in the kidney diet. For your wellbeing, you diversify your diet with low salt and low salt foods, which can have enough protein without raising your salt intake.

Brown rice contains a lot of phosphorus and potassium, so it can be eaten in small amounts and restricted in kidney foods. To prevent high dietary intake of potassium and phosphorus, the only way to fit brown rice into a kidney diet is to monitor the portion size and combine it with other foods. It's tough to get enough of the vitamins and nutrients you need after eating kidney-friendly meals.

If you have been diagnosed with chronic kidney disease (CKD), the phosphorus and calcium levels can need to be monitored and controlled. Electrolytes, nutrients, and liquids in the body are all balanced in this way. To keep the ratios of these electrolytes, minerals, and fluids in the body in check, people with kidney disease may need to limit their consumption of the following ingredients.

A person's dietary requirements can change if they have kidney disease, depending on how much residual kidney function there is, among other factors. For example, you can prescribe a high-protein diet for dialysis patients, but a low-protein diet for patients with chronic kidney disease. Since vegetarian protein sources include differing levels of potassium and phosphorus, a vegetarian kidney diet includes a bespoke diet from a certified dietitian.

BREAKFAST

1. Breakfast Smoothie

Preparation Time: 15 minutes

Cooking Time: 0 minutes

Servings: 2

Ingredients:

- Frozen blueberries – 1 cup
- Pineapple chunks – 1/2 cup
- English cucumber – 1/2 cup
- Apple – 1/2
- Water – 1/2 cup

Directions:

1. Put the pineapple, blueberries, cucumber, apple, and water in a blender and blend until thick and smooth.
2. Pour into 2 glasses and serve.

Nutrition: Calories: 87 Fat: g Carb: 22g Phosphorus: 28mg Potassium: 192mg Sodium: 3mg Protein: 0.7g

2. Salad with Vinaigrette

Preparation Time: 25 minutes

Cooking Time: 0 minutes

Servings: 4

Ingredients:

- For the vinaigrette:
- Olive oil – 1/2 cup
- Balsamic vinegar - 4 Tbsps.
- Chopped fresh oregano – 2 Tbsps.
- Pinch red pepper flakes
- Ground black pepper
- For the salad
- Shredded green leaf lettuce – 4 cups
- Carrot – 1, shredded
- Fresh green beans – ¾ cup, cut into 1-inch pieces
- Large radishes – 3, sliced thin

Directions:

1. To make the vinaigrette: put the vinaigrette Ingredients in a bowl and whisk.
2. To make the salad, in a bowl, toss together the carrot, lettuce, green beans, and radishes.
3. Add the vinaigrette to the vegetables and toss to coat.
4. Arrange the salad on plates and serve.

Nutrition: Calories: 273 Fat: 27g Carb: 7g Phosphorus: 30mg Potassium: 197mg Sodium: 27mg Protein: 1g

3. Salad with Lemon Dressing

Preparation Time: 10 minutes

Cooking Time: 0 minutes

Servings: 4

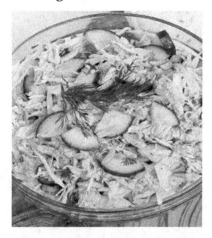

Ingredients:

- Heavy cream – 1/4 cup
- Freshly squeezed lemon juice – 1/4 cup
- Granulated sugar – 2 Tbsps.
- Chopped fresh dill – 2 Tbsps.
- Finely chopped scallion – 2 Tbsps. green part only
- Ground black pepper – 1/4 tsp.
- English cucumber – 1, sliced thin
- Shredded green cabbage – 2 cups

Directions:

1. In a small bowl, stir together the lemon juice, cream, sugar, dill, scallion, and pepper until well blended.

2. In a large bowl, toss together the cucumber and cabbage.

3. Place the salad in the refrigerator and chill for 1 hour.

4. Stir before serving.

Nutrition: Calories: 99 Fat: 6g Carb: 13g Phosphorus: 38mg Potassium: 200mg Sodium: 14mg Protein: 2g

4. Shrimp with Salsa

Preparation Time: 15 minutes

Cooking Time: 10 minutes

Servings: 4

Ingredients:

- Olive oil – 2 Tbsp.
- Large shrimp – 6 ounces, peeled and deveined, tails left on
- Minced garlic – 1 tsp.
- Chopped English cucumber – 1/2 cup
- Chopped mango – 1/2 cup
- Zest of 1 lime
- Juice of 1 lime
- Ground black pepper
- Lime wedges for garnish

Directions:

1. Soak 4 wooden skewers in water for 30 minutes.
2. Preheat the barbecue to medium heat.
3. In a bowl, toss together the olive oil, shrimp, and garlic.
4. Thread the shrimp onto the skewers, about 4 shrimp per skewer.

5. In a bowl, stir together the mango, cucumber, lime zest, and lime juice, and season the salsa lightly with pepper. Set aside.

6. Grill the shrimp for 10 minutes, turning once or until the shrimp is opaque and cooked through.

7. Season the shrimp lightly with pepper.

8. Serve the shrimp on the cucumber salsa with lime wedges on the side.

Nutrition: Calories: 120 Fat: 8g Carb: 4g Phosphorus: 91mg Potassium: 129mg Sodium: 60mg Protein: 9g

5. Pesto Pork Chops

Preparation Time: 20 minutes

Cooking Time: 20 minutes

Servings: 4

Ingredients:

- Pork top-loin chops – 4 (3-ounce) boneless, fat trimmed
- Herb pesto – 8 tsps.
- Breadcrumbs – 1/2 cup
- Olive oil – 1 Tbsp.

Directions:

1. Preheat the oven to 450F.
2. Line a baking sheet with foil. Set aside.
3. Rub 1 tsp. of pesto evenly over both sides of each pork chop.
4. Lightly dredge each pork chop in the breadcrumbs.
5. Heat the oil in a skillet.
6. Brown the pork chops on each side for 5 minutes.
7. Place the pork chops on the baking sheet.
8. Bake for 10 minutes or until pork reaches 145F in the center.

Nutrition: Calories: 210 Fat: 7g Carb: 10g Phosphorus: 179mg Potassium: 220mg Sodium: 148mg Protein: 24g

6. Turkey Burgers

Preparation Time: 15 minutes

Cooking Time: 8 minutes

Servings: 5

Ingredients:

- 1 ripe pear, peeled, cored and chopped roughly
- 1-pound lean ground turkey
- 1 teaspoon fresh ginger, grated finely
- 2 minced garlic cloves
- 1 teaspoon fresh rosemary, minced
- 1 teaspoon fresh sage, minced
- Salt, to taste
- Freshly ground black pepper, to taste
- 1-2 tablespoons coconut oil

Directions:

1. In a blender, add pear and pulse till smooth.
2. Transfer the pear mixture in a large bowl with remaining ingredients except for oil and mix till well combined.
3. Make small equal sized 10 patties from the mixture.
4. In a heavy-bottomed frying pan, heat oil on medium heat.
5. Add the patties and cook for around 4-5 minutes.
6. Flip the inside and cook for approximately 2-3 minutes.

Nutrition: Calories: 477 Fat: 15g Carbohydrates: 26g Fiber: 11g Protein: 35g

7. Collard Greens Dish

Preparation Time: 10 minutes

Cooking Time: 60 minutes

Servings: 6

Ingredients:

- 1 tablespoon olive oil
- 3 slices of bacon, sliced
- 1 large onion, chopped
- 2 garlic cloves, minced
- 1 teaspoon salt
- 3 cups chicken broth
- 1 red pepper flake
- 1-pound fresh collard greens, cut into 2-inch pieces

Directions:

1. Take a large-sized pan
2. Put oil and allow the oil to heat it up
3. Add bacon and cook it until crispy and remove it, crumble the bacon and add the crumbled bacon to the pan
4. Add onion and keep cooking for 5 minutes
5. Add garlic and cook until you have a nice fragrance
6. Add collard greens and keep frying until wilted, add chicken broth and season with pepper, salt, and red pepper flakes

7. Lessening the heat and cover with a lid, simmer for 45 minutes

8. Enjoy!

Nutrition: Calories: 127 Fat: 10g Carbohydrates: 8g Protein: 4g

8. Colorful Bean Salad

Preparation Time: 11 minutes

Cooking Time: 0 minute

Serving: 4

Ingredients:

- 200 g green beans
- 1 onion
- 1 bell pepper
- 1 small can (drained weight 250 g) white beans
- 1 small can (drained weight 250 g) kidney beans
- 2 tbsp wine vinegar
- 2 tbsp sour cream
- 1/2 teaspoon mustard
- 1/2 teaspoon tomato ketchup
- 1/2 teaspoon horseradish
- salt
- pepper
- 1 tbsp oil
- chopped thyme

Direction:

1. Clean and wash the green beans and cook in salted boiling water for 6-8 minutes until they are firm to the

bite. Pour into a sieve, rinse in cold water and drain well. Transfer to a large bowl.

2. Skin the onion and cut into thin rings. Halve and core the peppers lengthways, wash and cut into cubes. Drain the kidney beans and white beans each into a sieve, rinse with cold water and drain well. Then add the onion, bell pepper, kidney beans, and white beans to the green beans.

3. For the dressing mix together vinegar, sour cream, mustard, tomato ketchup, horseradish, oil, and thyme, season with salt and pepper. Mix with the salad ingredients and let the bean salad steep for about 5 minutes before serving.

Nutrition: 210 calories 7g protein 29mg potassium 132mg sodium

LUNCH

9. Roasted Cod with Plums

Preparation Time: 10 minutes

Cooking Time:20 minutes

Servings: 4

Ingredients:

- 6 red plums, halved and pitted
- 1½ pounds cod fillets
- 3 tablespoons extra-virgin olive oil
- 2 tablespoons freshly squeezed lemon juice
- ½ teaspoon dried thyme leaves
- 1/8 teaspoon salt
- 1/8 teaspoon freshly ground black pepper
- ¾ cup plain whole-almond milk yogurt, for serving

Directions:

1. Preheat the oven to 375°F. Line a baking sheet with parchment paper.
2. Arrange the plums, cut-side up, along with the fish on the prepared baking sheet. Drizzle with the olive oil and lemon juice and sprinkle with the thyme, salt, and pepper.
3. Roast for 15 to 20 minutes or until the fish flakes when tested with a fork and the plums are tender.
4. Serve with the yogurt.

5. Ingredient Tip: There's no need to measure out exactly 2 tablespoons of lemon juice. A standard-size lemon has approximately 2 tablespoons juice in it. Simply squeeze all the juice from the lemon, being careful to avoid squeezing in the seeds.

Nutrition: Calories: 230; Total fat: 9g; Saturated fat: 2g; Sodium: 154mg; Phosphorus: 197mg; Potassium: 437mg; Carbohydrates: 10g; Protein: 27g; Sugar: 8g

10. Lemon Chicken

Preparation Time: 20 minutes

Cooking Time: 24 minutes

Servings: 4

Ingredients:

- 2 lemons
- 12 ounces' boneless skinless chicken breasts, cubed
- 2 tablespoons extra-virgin olive oil
- 1/8 teaspoon salt
- 1/8 teaspoon freshly ground black pepper
- ½ large onion, chopped
- 1 cup 2-inch green bean pieces
- 1 cup 2-inch asparagus pieces

Directions:

1. Zest one of the lemons and place the zest into a medium bowl. Juice that lemon and add the juice to the bowl. Slice the remaining lemon, remove the seeds, and set aside.
2. In the bowl with the lemon juice, place the cubed chicken and set aside for 10 minutes to marinate.
3. When ready to cook, in a large skillet, heat the olive oil over medium heat.
4. Using a slotted spoon, remove the chicken from the lemon juice, reserving the lemon juice mixture. Add the chicken to the pan and cook for 3 to 4 minutes, stirring, until the chicken is lightly browned. It doesn't have to

be completely cooked. Transfer the chicken to a clean plate and sprinkle with the salt and pepper.

5. Add the sliced lemon to the skillet and cook for 3 minutes on each side, turning once, until it is slightly caramelized. Transfer to the plate with the chicken.

6. Add the onion to the skillet and cook for 3 to 4 minutes, until the onion is tender-crisp, stirring to loosen the chicken drippings from the skillet.

7. Add the green beans and sauté for 2 minutes. Add the asparagus and sauté for 1 minute.

8. Return the chicken to the skillet and add the reserved lemon juice. Simmer for 4 to 6 minutes or until the chicken is thoroughly cooked to 165°F, the vegetables are tender, and the sauce has slightly thickened.

9. Add the caramelized lemon slices to the skillet and cook for 1 to 2 minutes, stirring, until hot. Serve.

Nutrition: Calories: 207; Total fat: 9g; Saturated fat: 1g; Sodium: 121mg; Phosphorus: 245mg; Potassium: 593mg; Carbohydrates: 11g; Fiber: 4g; Protein: 22g; Sugar: 5g

11. **Curried Chicken Stir-Fry**

Preparation Time: 20 minutes

Cooking Time: 15 minutes

Servings: 6

Ingredients:

- 12 ounces' boneless skinless chicken breasts, cut into 1-inch cubes
- 2 teaspoons curry powder
- 1/8 teaspoon salt
- 1/8 teaspoon freshly ground black pepper
- 1 (20-ounce) can pineapple tidbits, strained, reserving juice
- 2 tablespoons extra-virgin olive oil
- 1 yellow onion, chopped
- 2 red bell peppers, chopped

Directions:

1. In a medium bowl, toss the chicken, curry powder, salt, and pepper and set aside.
2. In a small saucepan, heat the reserved pineapple juice over low heat. Let it reduce, stirring occasionally, while you make the rest of the stir-fry.
3. In a large skillet, heat the olive oil over medium heat. Add the chicken. Stir-fry for 3 for 4 minutes or until the chicken is light brown; it doesn't have to cook completely. Transfer the chicken to a plate.

4. Add the onion to the skillet and cook for 3 minutes, stirring, until the onion is crisp-tender. Check to make sure the pineapple liquid isn't burning and continue to stir it. Add the bell peppers and stir-fry for another 3 minutes, until crisp tender.

5. Return the chicken to the skillet, add the pineapple tidbits and cook, stirring, for 3 to 4 minutes or until the chicken is cooked through.

6. Add the thickened pineapple juice to the skillet and stir. Serve.

7. Increase Protein Tip: To make this a high-protein recipe, increase the chicken to 1 pound. The protein content will increase to 25g per serving.

Nutrition: Calories: 215; Total fat: 7g; Saturated fat: 1g; Sodium: 98mg; Phosphorus: 146mg; Potassium: 374mg; Carbohydrates: 19g; Fiber: 2g; Protein: 19g; Sugar: 16g

12. Thai-Style Chicken Salad

Preparation Time: 15 minutes

Cooking Time: 10 minutes

Servings: 6

Ingredients:

- 3 cups shredded cooked chicken (about 1 pound)
- 1 (10-ounce) package shredded cabbage with carrots
- 2 limes
- 1/3 cup extra-virgin olive oil
- ¼ cup peanut butter
- ¼ teaspoon freshly ground black pepper
- ¼ cup chopped peanuts

Directions:

1. In a large bowl, combine the chicken and cabbage and toss to mix.
2. In a small bowl, zest one of the limes. Juice both of the limes into the bowl. Add the olive oil, peanut butter, and pepper and mix with a whisk.
3. Drizzle the dressing over the salad and toss. Top with the peanuts and serve.
4. Ingredient Tip: If you like spicy food, add 1 or 2 minced jalapeño peppers to this salad. You could also add minced chipotle peppers in adobo sauce; just a teaspoon of each will add lots of heat.

Nutrition: Calories: 415; Total fat: 31g; Saturated fat: 5g; Sodium: 119mg; Phosphorus: 239mg; Potassium: 408mg; Carbohydrates: 9g; Fiber: 3g; Protein: 28g; Sugar: 3g

DINNER

13. Golden Eggplant Fries

Preparation Time: 10 minutes

Cooking Time: 15 minutes

Servings: 8

Ingredients:

- 2 eggs
- 2 cups almond flour
- 2 tablespoons coconut oil, spray
- 2 eggplant, peeled and cut thinly
- Sunflower seeds and pepper

Directions:

1. Preheat your oven to 400 degrees F.
2. Take a bowl and mix with sunflower seeds and black pepper.
3. Take another bowl and beat eggs until frothy.
4. Dip the eggplant pieces into the eggs.
5. Then coat them with the flour mixture.
6. Add another layer of flour and egg.
7. Then, take a baking sheet and grease with coconut oil on top.
8. Bake for about 15 minutes.

9. Serve and enjoy!

Nutrition: Calories: 212 Fat: 15.8g Carbohydrates: 12.1g Protein: 8.6g Phosphorus: 150mg Potassium: 147mg Sodium: 105mg

14. Very Wild Mushroom Pilaf

Preparation Time: 10 minutes

Cooking Time: 3 hours

Servings: 4

Ingredients:

- 1 cup wild rice
- 2 garlic cloves, minced
- 6 green onions, chopped
- 2 tablespoons olive oil
- ½ pound baby Bella mushrooms
- 2 cups water

Directions:

1. Add rice, garlic, onion, oil, mushrooms and water to your Slow Cooker.
2. Stir well until mixed.
3. Place lid and cook on LOW for 3 hours.
4. Stir pilaf and divide between serving platters.
5. Enjoy!

Nutrition: Calories: 210 Fat: 7g Carbohydrates: 16g Protein: 4g Phosphorus: 110mg Potassium: 117mg Sodium: 75mg

15. Sporty Baby Carrots

Preparation Time: 5 minutes

Cooking Time: 5 minutes

Servings: 4

Ingredients:

- 1-pound baby carrots
- 1 cup water
- 1 tablespoon clarified ghee
- 1 tablespoon chopped up fresh mint leaves
- Sea flavored vinegar as needed

Directions:

1. Place a steamer rack on top of your pot and add the carrots.
2. Add water.
3. Lock the lid and cook at HIGH pressure for 2 minutes.
4. Do a quick release.
5. Pass the carrots through a strainer and drain them.
6. Wipe the insert clean.
7. Return the insert to the pot and set the pot to Sauté mode.
8. Add clarified butter and allow it to melt.
9. Add mint and sauté for 30 seconds.
10. Add carrots to the insert and sauté well.

11. Remove them and sprinkle with bit of flavored vinegar on top.

12. Enjoy!

Nutrition: Calories: 131 Fat: 10g Carbohydrates: 11g Protein: 1g Phosphorus: 130mg Potassium: 147mg Sodium: 85mg

MAIN DISHES

16. Savory Bread

Preparation Time: 10 minutes

Cooking Time: 20-25 minutes

Servings: 8-10

Ingredients:

- ½ cup plus 1tablespoon almond flour
- 1 tsp. baking soda
- 1 teaspoon ground turmeric
- Salt, to taste
- 2 large organic eggs
- 2 organic egg whites
- 1 cup raw cashew butter
- 1 tablespoon water
- 1 tablespoon apple cider vinegar

Directions:

1. Set the oven to 350F. Grease a loaf pan.
2. In a big pan, mix together flour, baking soda, turmeric, and salt.
3. In another bowl, add eggs, egg whites, and cashew butter and beat till smooth.
4. Gradually, add water and beat till well combined.
5. Add flour mixture and mix till well combined.
6. Stir in apple cider vinegar treatment.

7. Place a combination into prepared loaf pan evenly.
8. Bake for around twenty minutes or till a toothpick inserted within the center is released clean.

Nutrition: Calories: 347 Fat: 11g Carbohydrates: 29g Fiber: 6g Protein: 21g

17. Savory Veggie Muffins

Preparation Time: 15 minutes

Cooking Time: 18-23 minutes

Servings: 5

Ingredients:

- ¾ cup almond meal
- ½ tsp baking soda
- ¼ cup concentrate powder
- 2 teaspoons fresh dill, chopped
- Salt, to taste
- 4 large organic eggs
- 1½ tablespoons nutritional yeast
- 2 teaspoons apple cider vinegar
- 3 tablespoons fresh lemon juice
- 2 tablespoons coconut oil, melted
- 1 cup coconut butter, softened
- 1 bunch scallion, chopped
- 2 medium carrots, peeled and grated
- ½ cup fresh parsley, chopped

Directions:

1. Set the oven to 350F. Grease 10 cups of your large muffin tin.
2. In a large bowl, mix together flour, baking soda, Protein powder, and salt.
3. In another bowl, add eggs, nutritional yeast, vinegar, lemon juice, and oil and beat till well combined.

4. Add coconut butter and beat till the mixture becomes smooth.
5. Put egg mixture into the flour mixture and mix till well combined.
6. Fold in scallion, carts, and parsley.
7. Place the amalgamation into prepared muffin cups evenly.
8. Bake for about 18-23 minutes or till a toothpick inserted inside center comes out clean.

Nutrition: Calories: 378 Fat: 13g Carbohydrates: 32g Fiber: 11g Protein: 32g

18. Crepes with Coconut Cream & Strawberry Sauce

Preparation Time: 15 minutes

Cooking Time: 8 minutes

Servings: 4

Ingredients:

- For Sauce:
- 12-ounces frozen strawberries, thawed and liquid reserved
- 1½ teaspoons tapioca starch
- 1 tablespoon honey
- For the Coconut cream:
- 1 (13½-ounce) can chilled coconut almond milk
- 1 teaspoon organic vanilla flavoring
- 1 tablespoon organic honey
- For Crepes:
- 2 tablespoons tapioca starch
- 2 tablespoons coconut flour
- ¼ cup almond milk
- 2 organic eggs
- Pinch of salt
- Almond oil, as required

Directions:

1. For sauce inside a bowl, mix together some reserved strawberry liquid and tapioca starch.
2. Add remaining ingredients and mix well.

3. Transfer a combination inside a pan on medium-high heat.
4. Bring to a boil, stirring continuously.
5. Cook for at least 2-3 minutes, till the sauce, becomes thick.
6. Remove from heat and aside, covered till serving.
7. For coconut cream, carefully, scoop your cream from your surface of a can of coconut almond milk.
8. In a mixer, add coconut cream, vanilla flavoring, and honey and pulse for around 6-8 minutes or till fluffy.
9. For crepes in a blender, add all ingredients and pulse till well combined and smooth.
10. Lightly, grease a substantial nonstick skillet with almond oil as well as heat on medium-low heat.
11. Add a modest amount of mixture and tilt the pan to spread it evenly inside the skillet.
12. Cook approximately 1-2 minutes.
13. Carefully change the side and cook for approximately 1-1½ minutes more.
14. Repeat with the remaining mixture.
15. Divide the coconut cream onto each crepe evenly and fold into quarters.
16. Place strawberry sauce ahead and serve.

Nutrition: Calories: 364 Fat: 9g Carbohydrates: 26g Fiber: 7g Protein: 15g

SNACKS

19. Hummus with Celery

Preparation Time: 15 minutes

Cooking Time: 0 minutes

Servings: 4

Ingredients:

- 1/4 cup lemon juice
- 1/4 cup tahini
- 3 cloves of garlic, crushed
- 2 tablespoons extra virgin olive oil
- 1/2 teaspoon salt
- 1/2 teaspoon cumin
- 1 (15–ounce) can chickpeas
- 2 to 3 tablespoons water
- Dash of paprika
- 6 stalks celery, cut into 2-inch pieces
- 3 tablespoons salsa

Directions:

1. Using a food processor mix the lemon juice and tahini for about a minute, until it is smooth. Scrape the sides down and process for 30 more seconds.
2. Add the garlic, olive oil, salt, and cumin. Blend for about 1 minute.

3. Drain the chickpeas, put the half of them on the food processor, and blend for another minute. Scrape down the sides, add the other half of the chickpeas, and process until smooth, about 2 minutes. If it like a little too thick, add water, 1 tablespoon at a time until you reach the desired consistency.
4. Fill the celery sticks with hummus and sprinkle paprika on top.
5. Serve with salsa for dipping.

Nutrition: Calories: 240 kcal Protein: 9.27 g Fat: 14.51 g Carbohydrates: 21.01 g

20. Lemony Ginger Cookies

Preparation Time: 15 minutes + 30 minutes chill time

Cooking Time: 10-12 minutes

Servings: 25

Ingredients:

- 1/2 cup arrowroot flour
- 1 1/2 cups stevia
- 3/4 teaspoon salt
- 1/2 teaspoon baking soda
- 1 teaspoon nutritional yeast
- 3 inches of ginger root, peeled and diced
- 1 1/2 cup coconut butter, softened
- Zest of 1 lemon
- 2 teaspoons vanilla

Directions:

1. Set the oven to 350F, then line two or three cookie sheets with parchment paper.
2. Mix the arrowroot flour, stevia, salt, soda, and yeast in a bowl.
3. In another bowl, put the remaining ingredients and mix well.
4. Put in the dry ingredients gradually until well combined. If the dough is too soft, put an additional 1 to 2 tablespoons of arrowroot powder. The dough will stiffen when chilled, so be careful.

5. Wrap the dough in parchment and press it flat. Chill for 30 minutes.
6. Take a chunk of the chilled dough and flatten it between two pieces of parchment until it is 1/8 inch thick. Dust with a little arrowroot powder and cut into shapes.
7. Place on baking sheets about 1 inch apart and bake 10 to 12 minutes. Cool on cookie sheets for 15 minutes before removing.

Nutrition: Calories: 112 kcal Protein: 0.44 g Fat: 11.3 g Carbohydrates: 2.49 g

21. **Mandarin Cottage Cheese**

Preparation Time: 5 minutes

Cooking Time: 0 minutes

Servings: 1

Ingredients:

- 1/2 cup low-fat cottage cheese
- 1/2 cup canned mandarin mangos
- 1 1/2 tablespoons slivered almonds

Directions:

1. Place the cottage cheese in a bowl.
2. Drain the mandarin mangos, place them atop the cottage cheese, and sprinkle with almonds.

Nutrition: Calories: 360 kcal Protein: 26.24 g Fat: 21.37 g Carbohydrates: 15.22 g

22. Mushroom Chips

Preparation Time: 10 minutes

Cooking Time: 45-60 minutes

Servings: 2-4

Ingredients:

- 16 ounces of king oyster mushrooms
- 2 tablespoons ghee
- Kosher salt and ground pepper to taste

Directions:

1. Set the oven to 300F, then line two cookie sheets with parchment paper.
2. Cut every mushroom in half lengthwise, then cut with a mandolin into 1/8 inch slices or strips. Place them on cookie sheets with some room in between. Melt the ghee and brush it over the mushrooms, then season with the salt and pepper.
3. Bake for at least 45 minutes to 1 hour, until they are completely crisp. Store in airtight containers.

Nutrition: Calories: 62 kcal Protein: 5.58 g Fat: 2 g Carbohydrates: 7.97 g

23. **Toasted Pumpkin Seeds**

Preparation Time: 5 minutes

Cooking Time: 30 minutes

Servings:2-4

Ingredients:

- 1 to 2 cups pumpkin seeds
- Water
- 1 teaspoon salt
- 1/2 teaspoon extra virgin olive oil
- Sea salt

Directions:

1. Put seeds in a saucepan and cover with water. Add salt.
2. Bring it to a boil and boil for 10 minutes.
3. Simmer uncovered for 10 more minutes. This makes the seeds very crispy when baked. Drain the seeds and pat dry using a paper towel.
4. Cover a baking sheet with parchment paper and spread out the seeds in a single layer.
5. Dust with salt, then bake in an oven at 325F for at least 10 minutes, stirring halfway through.
6. Cool, then store in an airtight container.

Nutrition: Calories: 192 kcal Protein: 10.41 g Fat: 16.23 g Carbohydrates: 4.34 g

24. Easy Black and White Brownies

Preapration Time:10 minutes

Cooking Time:: 20 minutes

Servings: 1 dozen brownies

Ingredients:

- 1 egg
- 1/4cup brown sugar
- 2 tablespoons white sugar
- 2 tablespoons safflower oil
- 1 teaspoon vanilla
- 1/3cup all-purpose flour
- 1/4cup cocoa powder
- 1/4cup white chocolate chips
- Nonstick cooking spray

Directions:

1. Spritz a baking pan with nonstick cooking spray.
2. Whisk together the egg, white sugar, and brown sugar in a medium bowl. Mix in the vanilla and safflower oil and stir to combine.
3. Add the cocoa powder and flour and stir just until incorporated. Fold in the white chocolate chips.
4. Scrape the batter into the Directions:ared baking pan.
5. Place the pan on the bake position.
6. Select bake, set temperature to 340ºf (171ºc), and set Time to 20 minutes.

7. When done, the brownie should spring back when touched lightly with your fingers.

8. Transfer to a wire rack and let cool for 30 minutes before slicing to serve.

Nutrition: Calories 68 Fat 6.1 g Carbohydrates 1.2 g Sugar 0.3 g Protein 3 g Cholesterol 0 mg

25. <u>Chocolate Brownie Bar</u>

Preapration Time:10 minutes

Cooking Time: 16 minutes

Servings:4

Ingredients:

- 1 cup bananas, overripe
- 1 scoop protein powder
- 2 tbsp unsweetened cocoa powder
- 1/2 cup almond butter, melted

Directions:

1. Preheat the air fryer to 325 f.
2. Spray air fryer baking pan with cooking spray.
3. Add all Ingredients:into the blender and blend until smooth.
4. Pour batter into the Directions:ared pan and place in the air fryer basket.
5. Cook brownie for 16 minutes.
6. Serve and enjoy.

Nutrition: Calories: 164 Protein: 2 g. Fat: 22 g. Carbs: 4 g.

26. <u>Brownies</u>

Preapration Time:10 minutes

Cooking Time: 20 minutes

Servings: 2

Ingredients:

- ¼ cup of all-purpose flour
- ¼ teaspoon baking powder
- 1/3 cup of cocoa powder
- ¼ cup of butter
- ½ cup of granulated sugar
- 1 egg, beaten Pinch salt

Directions:

1. Spray baking pan with oil.
2. In a bowl, mix all the Ingredients:.
3. Pour the mixture into the baking pan.
4. Set your air fryer to bake.
5. Cook at 350 degrees F for 18 to twenty minutes.
6. Serving Suggestions: Let cool for 10 minutes before slicing and serving.
7. Directions: & Cooking Tips: You'll also top the brownies with chopped walnuts.

Nutrition: Calories 68 Fat 6.1 g Carbohydrates 1.2 g Sugar 0.3 g Protein 3 g Cholesterol 0 mg

27. Easy Mug Brownie

Preapration Time:5 minutes

Cooking Time: 10 minutes

Servings:1

Ingredients:

- 1scoop chocolate protein powder
- 1tbsp cocoa powder
- 1/2 tsp baking powder
- 1/4 cup unsweetened almond milk

Directions:

1. Add baking powder, protein powder, and cocoa powder in a mug and mix well.
2. Add milk in a mug and stir well.
3. Place the mug in the air fryer and cook at 390 F for 10 minutes.
4. Serve and enjoy.

Nutrition: Calories 68 Fat 6.1 g Carbohydrates 1.2 g Sugar 0.3 g Protein 3 g Cholesterol 0 mg

28. Brownie Bites

Preapration Time:10 minutes

Cooking Time: 12 minutes

Servings:16

Ingredients:

- ¾ cup almond flour
- ½ tsp vanilla
- 2 eggs
- ½ cup unsweetened cocoa powder
- ¾ cup swerve
- 4 tbsp butter, melted Pinch of salt

Directions:

1. Preheat the air fryer to 325 F.
2. In a bowl, whisk together butter, vanilla, eggs, cocoa powder, sweetener, and salt.
3. Add almond flour and stir to combine.
4. Pour batter into the mini silicone molds and place into the air fryer.
5. Cook for 12 minutes or until done.
6. Serve and enjoy.

Nutrition: calories: 181 protein: 3 g. Fat: 98 g. Carbs: 42 g.

29. <u>Yummy Brownies</u>

Preapration Time:10 minutes

Cooking Time: 10 minutes

Servings:4

- **Ingredients**:
- 2tbsp cocoa powder
- 1/4 tsp baking powder
- 1/2 tsp baking soda
- 2tbsp unsweetened applesauce
- 1tsp liquid stevia
- 1tbsp coconut oil, melted
- 3tbsp almond flour
- 1/2 tsp vanilla
- 1tbsp unsweetened almond milk
- 1/2 cup almond butter
- 1/4 tsp sea salt

Directions:

1. Preheat the air fryer to 350 F.
2. Grease air fryer baking dish with cooking spray and set aside.
3. In a small bowl, mix together almond flour, baking soda, cocoa powder, baking powder, and salt. Set aside.
4. In a small bowl, add coconut oil and almond butter and microwave until melted.
5. Add sweetener, vanilla, almond milk, and applesauce in the coconut oil mixture and stir well.

6. Add dry Ingredients:to the wet Ingredients:and stir to combine.
7. Pour batter into Directions:ared dish and place into the air fryer and cook for 10 minutes.
8. Slice and serve.

Nutrition: calories: 185 protein: 4 g. Fat: 88 g. Carbs: 32 g.

30. __Almond Bars__

Preapration Time:10 minutes

Cooking Time: 35 minutes

Servings:12

Ingredients:

- 2 eggs, lightly beaten
- 1cup erythritol
- ½ tsp vanilla
- ¼ cup water
- ½ cup butter, softened
- ¾ cup cherries, pitted 1 ½ cup almond flour
- 1tbsp xanthan gum
- ½tsp salt

Directions:

1. In a bowl, mix together almond flour, erythritol, eggs, vanilla, butter, and salt until dough is formed.
2. Press dough in air fryer baking dish.
3. Place in the air fryer and cook at 375 F for 10 minutes.
4. Meanwhile, mix together cherries, xanthan gum, and water.
5. Pour cherry mixture over cooked dough and cook for 25 minutes more.
6. Slice and serve.

Nutrition: calories: 181 protein: 3 g. Fat: 98 g. Carbs: 42 g.

31. Chocolate Vanilla Bars

Preapration Time:10 Minutes

Cooking Time: 7 Minutes

Servings: 12

Ingredients:

- 1 cup sugar free and vegan chocolate chips
- 2tablespoons coconut butter
- 2/3 cup coconut cream
- tablespoons stevia
- ¼ teaspoon vanilla extract

Directions:

1. Put the cream in a bowl, add stevia, butter and chocolate chips and stir
2. Leave aside for 5 minutes, stir well and mix the vanilla.
3. Transfer the mix into a lined baking sheet, introduce in your air fryer and cook at 356 degrees F for 7 minutes.
4. Leave the mix aside to cool down, slice and serve. Enjoy!

Nutrition: Calories: 120 Protein: 1 g. Fat: 5 g. Carbs: 6 g.

32. <u>Raspberry Bars</u>

Preapration Time:10 Minutes

Cooking Time: 6 Minutes

Servings: 12

Ingredients:

- 1/2 cup coconut butter, melted
- 1/2 cup coconut oil
- 1/2 cup raspberries, dried
- ¼ cup swerve
- 1/2 cup coconut, shredded

Directions:

1. In your food processor, blend dried berries very well.
2. In a bowl that fits your air fryer, mix oil with butter, swerve, coconut and raspberries, toss well, introduce in the fryer and cook at 320 degrees F for 6 minutes.
3. Spread this on a lined baking sheet, keep in the fridge for an hour, slice and serve.
4. Enjoy!

Nutrition: Calories: 164 Protein: 2 g. Fat: 22 g. Carbs: 4 g.

33. Oat Chocolate Cookies

Preapration Time:10 Minutes

Cooking Time:: 20 Minutes

Servings: 8

Ingredients:

- 1 cup unsalted butter, at room temperature
- 1 cup dark brown sugar
- ½ cup granulated sugar
- 2 large eggs
- 1 tablespoon vanilla extract
- Pinch salt
- 2 cups old-fashioned rolled oats
- 1½ cups all-purpose flour
- 1 teaspoon baking powder
- 1 teaspoon baking soda
- 2 cups chocolate chips

Directions:

1. Stir together the butter, granulated sugar, and brown sugar in a large mixing bowl until smooth and light in color.
2. Crack the eggs into the bowl, one at a Time, mixing after each addition. Stir in the vanilla and salt.
3. Mix together the oats, flour, baking soda, and baking powder in a separate bowl. Add the mixture to the butter mixture and stir until mixed. Stir in the chocolate chips.

4. Spread the dough onto the sheet pan in an even layer.
5. Place the basket on the bake position.
6. Select bake, set temperature to 350ºf (180ºc), and set Time to 20 minutes.
7. After 15 minutes, check the cookie, rotating the pan if the crust is not browning evenly. Continue cooking for a total of 18 to 20 minutes or until golden brown.
8. When cooking is complete, remove the pan from the air fryer grill and allow to cool completely before slicing and serving.

Nutrition: Calories: 184 Protein: 9 g. Fat: 6 g. Carbs: 24 g.

SOUP AND STEW

34. Sweet Potato and Corn Soup

Preparation Time: 10 minutes

Cooking Time: 20 minutes

Servings: 4

Ingredients:

- ¼ cup extra-virgin olive oil or coconut oil
- 1 medium zucchini, cut into ¼-inch dice
- 1 cup broccoli florets
- 1 cup thinly sliced mushrooms
- 1 small onion, cut into ¼-inch dice
- 4 cups vegetable broth
- 2 cups peeled carrots cut into ¼-inch dice
- 1 cup frozen corn kernels
- 1 cup coconut almond milk or almond milk
- 2 tablespoons finely chopped fresh flat-leaf parsley
- 1 teaspoon salt
- ¼ teaspoon freshly ground black pepper

Directions:

1. In a huge pot, heat the oil on high heat.
2. Add the zucchini, broccoli, mushrooms, and onion and sauté until softened, 5 to 8 minutes.
3. Pour the broth and carrots and place it to a boil.

4. Reduce the heat to a simmer and cook until the carrots are tender, 5 to 7 minutes.

5. Add the corn, coconut almond milk, parsley, salt, and pepper. Cook on low heat up to the corn is heated through and serve.

Nutrition: Calories: 402 Total Fat: 29g Total Carbohydrates: 31g Sugar: 9g Fiber: 6g Protein: 10g Sodium: 1406mg

35. Chickpea Curry Soup

Preparation Time: 10 minutes

Cooking Time: 25 minutes

Servings: 4

Ingredients:

- ¼ cup extra-virgin olive oil or coconut oil
- 1 medium onion, finely chopped
- 2 garlic cloves, sliced
- 1 large apple, cored, peeled, and cut into ¼-inch dice
- 2 teaspoons curry powder
- 1 teaspoon salt
- 3 cups peeled butternut squash cut into ½-inch dice
- 3 cups vegetable broth
- 1 cup full-fat coconut almond milk
- 1 (15-ounce) can chickpeas, drained and rinsed
- 2 tablespoons finely chopped fresh cilantro

Directions:

1. In a huge pot, heat the oil on high heat.
2. Add the onion and garlic and sauté until the onion begins to brown, 6 to 8 minutes.
3. Put the apple, curry powder, and salt and sauté to toast the curry powder, 1 to 2 minutes.
4. Put the squash and broth then bring to a boil.
5. Lower the heat then cook until the squash is tender about 10 minutes.
6. Stir in the coconut almond milk.

7. Using an immersion blender, purée the soup in the pot until smooth.

8. Stir in the chickpeas and cilantro, heat through for 1 to 2 minutes, and serve.

Nutrition: Calories: 469 Total Fat: 30g Total Carbohydrates: 45g Sugar: 14g Fiber: 10g Protein: 12g Sodium: 1174mg

36. Onion, Kale and White Bean Soup

Preparation Time: 15 minutes

Cooking Time: 25 minutes

Servings: 4

Ingredients:

- ¼ cup extra-virgin olive oil
- 1 large onion, thinly sliced
- 2 garlic cloves, thinly sliced
- 1 teaspoon salt
- ¼ teaspoon freshly ground black pepper
- 1/8 Teaspoon red pepper flakes (optional)
- 3 cups stemmed kale leaves cut into ½-inch pieces
- 4 cups vegetable broth
- 1 (15½-ounce) can white beans, drained and rinsed
- 1 teaspoon finely chopped fresh rosemary

Directions:

1. In a huge pot, heat the oil on high heat.
2. Reduce the heat to medium, and add the onion, garlic, salt, pepper, and red pepper flakes (if using). Sauté until the onion is golden, about 10 minutes.
3. Add the kale, and sauté until wilted, 1 to 2 minutes.
4. Pour the broth then bring to a boil.
5. Reduce the heat to simmer, and cook until the kale is soft about 5 minutes.
6. Add the beans and rosemary. Cook until the beans are warmed through at least 2 to 3 minutes and serve.

Nutrition: Calories: 285 Total Fat: 15g Total Carbohydrates: 28g Sugar: 3g Fiber: 9g Protein: 13g Sodium: 1368mg

37. White rice and Shitake Miso Soup with Scallion

Preparation Time: 10 minutes

Cooking Time: 45 minutes

Servings: 4

Ingredients:

- 2 tablespoons sesame oil
- 1 cup thinly sliced shiitake mushroom caps
- 1 garlic clove, minced
- 1 (1½-inch) piece fresh ginger, peeled and sliced
- 1 cup medium-grain white rice
- ½ teaspoon salt
- 1 tablespoon white miso
- 2 scallions, thinly sliced
- 2 tablespoons finely chopped fresh cilantro

Directions:

1. In a huge pot, heat the oil on medium-high heat.
2. Add the mushrooms, garlic, and ginger and sauté until the mushrooms begin to soften, about 5 minutes.
3. Put the rice and stir to evenly coat with the oil.
4. Add 2 cups of water and salt and place it to a boil.
5. Lower the heat then cook until the rice is tender, 30 to 40 minutes.
6. Use a little of the soup broth to soften the miso, then stir it into the pot until well blended.
7. Mix in the scallions and cilantro, then serve.

Nutrition: Calories: 265 Total Fat: 8g Total Carbohydrates: 43g
Sugar: 2g Fiber: 3g Protein: 5g Sodium: 456mg

VEGETABLE

38. Pesto Pasta Salad

Preparation Time: 15 minutes

Cooking Time: 15 minutes

Servings: 4

Ingredients:

- 1 cup fresh basil leaves
- ½ cup packed fresh flat-leaf parsley leaves
- ½ cup arugula, chopped
- 2 tablespoons Parmesan cheese, grated
- ¼ cup extra-virgin olive oil
- 3 tablespoons mayonnaise
- 2 tablespoons water
- 12 ounces whole-wheat rotini pasta
- 1 red bell pepper, chopped
- 1 medium yellow summer squash, sliced
- 1 cup frozen baby peas

Directions:

1. Boil water in a large pot.
2. Meanwhile, combine the basil, parsley, arugula, cheese, and olive oil in a blender or food processor. Process

until the herbs are finely chopped. Add the mayonnaise and water, then process again. Set aside.

3. Prepare the pasta to the pot of boiling water; cook according to package directions, about 8 to 9 minutes. Drain well, reserving ¼ cup of the cooking liquid.

4. Combine the pesto, pasta, bell pepper, squash, and peas in a large bowl and toss gently, adding enough reserved pasta cooking liquid to make a sauce on the salad. Serve immediately or cover and chill, then serve.

5. Store covered in the refrigerator for up to 3 days.

Nutrition: Calories: 378 Fat: 24g Carbohydrates: 35g Protein: 9g Sodium: 163mg Potassium: 472mg Phosphorus: 213mg

39. Barley Blueberry Salad

Preparation Time: 15 minutes

Cooking Time: 15 minutes

Servings: 4

Ingredients:

- 1 cup quick-cooking barley
- 3 cups low-sodium vegetable broth
- 3 tablespoons extra-virgin olive oil
- 2 tablespoons freshly squeezed lemon juice
- 1 teaspoon yellow mustard
- 1 teaspoon honey
- 2 cups blueberries
- ¼ cup crumbled feta cheese

Directions:

1. Combine the barley and vegetable broth in a medium saucepan and bring to a simmer.

2. Reduce the heat to low, partially cover the pan, and simmer for 10 to 12 minutes or until the barley is tender.

3. Meanwhile, whisk together the olive oil, lemon juice, mustard, and honey in a serving bowl until blended.

4. Drain the barley if necessary and add to the bowl; toss to combine.

5. Add the blueberries, and feta and toss gently. Serve.

Nutrition: Calories: 345 Fat 16g Carbohydrates: 44gProtein: 7g
Sodium: 259mg Potassium: 301mg Phosphorus: 152mg

40. **Pasta with Creamy Broccoli Sauce**

Preparation Time: 15 minutes

Cooking Time: 15 minutes

Servings: 4

Ingredients:

- 2 tablespoons olive oil
- 1-pound broccoli florets
- 3 garlic cloves, halved
- 1 cup low-sodium vegetable broth
- ½ pound whole-wheat spaghetti pasta
- 4 ounces cream cheese
- 1 teaspoon dried basil leaves
- ½ cup grated Parmesan cheese

Directions:

1. Prepare a large pot of water to a boil.
2. Put olive oil in a large skillet. Sauté the broccoli and garlic for 3 minutes.
3. Add the broth to the skillet and bring to a simmer. Reduce the heat to low, partially cover the skillet, and simmer until the broccoli is tender about 5 to 6 minutes.
4. Cook the pasta according to package directions. Drain when al dente, reserving 1 cup pasta water.
5. When the broccoli is tender, add the cream cheese and basil—purée using an immersion blender.

6. Put mixture into a food processor, about half at a time, and purée until smooth and transfer the sauce back into the skillet.

7. Add the cooked pasta to the broccoli sauce. Toss, adding enough pasta water until the sauce coats the pasta completely. Sprinkle with the Parmesan and serve.

Nutrition: Calories: 302 Fat 14g Carbohydrates: 36g Protein: 11g Sodium: 260mg Potassium: 375mg Phosphorus: 223mg

SIDE DISHES

41. Broccoli and Almonds Mix

Preparation Time: 10 minutes

Cooking Time: 11 minutes

Servings: 4

Ingredients:

- 1 tablespoon olive oil
- 1 garlic clove, minced
- 1 pound broccoli florets
- 1/3 cup almonds, chopped
- Black pepper to taste

Directions:

1. Heat up a pan with the oil over medium-high heat, add the almonds, stir, cook for 5 minutes and transfer to a bowl,

2. Heat up the same pan again over medium-high heat, add broccoli and garlic, stir, cover and cook for 6 minutes more.

3. Add the almonds and black pepper to taste, stir, divide between plates and serve.

4. Enjoy!

Nutrition: Calories 116, fat 7,8, fiber 4, carbs 9,5, protein 4,9
Phosphorus: 110mg Potassium: 117mg Sodium: 75mg

42. Squash and Cranberries

Preparation Time: 10 minutes

Cooking Time: 30 minutes

Servings: 2

Ingredients:

- 1 tablespoon coconut oil
- 1 butternut squash, peeled and cubed
- 2 garlic cloves, minced
- 1 small yellow onion, chopped
- 12 ounces coconut almond milk
- 1 teaspoon curry powder
- 1 teaspoon cinnamon powder
- ½ cup cranberries

Directions:

1. Spread squash pieces on a lined baking sheet, place in the oven at 425 degrees F, bake for 15 minutes and leave to one side.
2. Heat up a pan with the oil over medium high heat, add garlic and onion, stir and cook for 5 minutes.
3. Add roasted squash, stir and cook for 3 minutes.
4. Add coconut almond milk, cranberries, cinnamon and curry powder, stir and cook for 5 minutes more.
5. Divide between plates and serve as a side dish!

6. Enjoy!

Nutrition: Calories 518, fat 47,6, fiber 7,3, carbs 24,9, protein 5,3 Phosphorus: 110mg Potassium: 117mg Sodium: 75mg

SALAD

43. Cucumber Salad

Preparation time:5 minutes

Cooking time:5 minutes

Servings:4

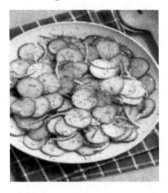

Ingredients:

- 1 tbsp. dried dill
- 1 onion
- ¼ cup water
- 1 cup vinegar
- 3 cucumbers
- ¾ cup white sugar

Direction:

1. In a bowl add all ingredients and mix well
2. Serve with dressing

Nutrition: Calories 49, Fat 0.1g, Sodium (Na) 341mg, Potassium (K) 171mg, Protein 0.8g, Carbs 11g, Phosphorus 24 mg

44. Tangy Glazed Black Cod

Preparation Time: 10 min

Cooking Time: 15 minutes

Servings: 4

Ingredients:

- 3 tablespoons fresh lime juice

- 2 tablespoons honey

- 2 tablespoons vinegar

- 1 tablespoon soy sauce

- 1 (1 pound) fillet black cod, bones removed

Directions:

1. Preheat oven to 425 degrees F. Spray the bottom of a Dutch oven or covered casserole dish with cooking spray.

2. Combine lime juice, honey, vinegar, and soy sauce in a saucepan over medium heat; cook and stir until sauce is thickened, about 5 minutes.

3. Place cod in the prepared Dutch oven. Pour sauce over fish Cover dish with an oven-safe lid.

4. Bake in the preheated oven until fish flakes easily with a fork, about 10 minutes.

Nutrition: Calories 44, Total Fat 0g, Saturated Fat 0g, Cholesterol 0mg, Sodium 127mg, Total Carbohydrate 11.8g, Dietary Fiber 0.2g, Total Sugars 9.3g, Protein 0.5g, Calcium 6mg, Iron 0mg, Potassium 58mg, Potassium 40mg

45. **Marinated Fried Fish**

Preparation Time: 15 min

Cooking Time: 10 minutes

Servings: 4

Ingredients:

- 2 (4 ounce) Salmon fillets
- 2 tablespoons lemon juice
- 2 tablespoons garlic powder
- 2 teaspoons ground cumin
- 1 teaspoon paprika
- 1/2 cup all-purpose flour
- 1 teaspoon dried rosemary
- 1/4 teaspoon cayenne pepper, or to taste
- 1 egg, beaten
- 1 tablespoon water
- ½ cup olive oil for frying

Directions:

1. Place salmon fillets in a small glass dish. Mix lemon juice, garlic powder, cumin, and paprika in a small bowl; pour over salmon fillets. Cover dish with plastic wrap and marinate salmon in refrigerator for 2 hours.

2. Mix flour, rosemary, and cayenne pepper together on a piece of waxed paper.

3. Beat egg and water together in a wide bowl.

4. Heat oil in a large skillet over medium heat.

5. Gently press the salmon fillets into the flour mixture to coat; shake to remove excess flour. Dip into the beaten egg to coat and immediately return to the flour mixture to coat.

6. Fry flounder in hot oil until the fish flakes easily with a fork, about 5 minutes per side.

Nutrition: Calories 139, Total Fat 4.7g, Saturated Fat 0.9g, Cholesterol 50mg, Sodium 30mg, Total Carbohydrate 16.3g, Dietary Fiber 1.4g, Total Sugars 1.4g, Protein 8.2g, Calcium 34mg, Iron 2mg, Potassium 203mg, Potassium 140mg

46. Spicy Lime and Basil Grilled Fish

Preparation Time: 30 min

Cooking Time: 30 minutes

Servings: 4

Ingredients:

- 2 pounds salmon fillets, each cut into thirds
- 6 tablespoons butter, melted
- 1 lime, juiced
- 1 tablespoon dried basil
- 1 teaspoon red pepper flakes
- 1 onion, sliced crosswise 1/8-inch thick

Directions:

1. Preheat grill for medium heat and lightly oil the grate.
2. Lay 4 8x10-inch pieces of aluminum foil onto a flat work surface and spray with cooking spray.
3. Arrange equal amounts of the salmon into the center of each foil square.
4. Stir butter, lime juice, basil, and red pepper flakes together in a small bowl; drizzle evenly over each portion of fish. Top each portion with onion slices.
5. Bring opposing ends of the foil together and roll together to form a seam. Roll ends toward fish to seal packets.

6. Cook packets on the preheated grill until fish flakes easily with a fork, 5 to 7 minutes per side.

Nutrition: Calories 151, Total Fat 13.4g, Saturated Fat 7.6g, Cholesterol 43mg, Sodium 95mg, Total Carbohydrate 3.1g, Dietary Fiber 0.8g, Total Sugars 1g, Protein 6g, Calcium 23mg, Iron 0mg, Potassium 158mg, Potassium 137mg

47. Steamed Fish with Garlic

Preparation Time: 15 min

Cooking Time: 45 minutes

Servings: 4

Ingredients:

- 2 (6 ounce) fillets cod fillets
- 3 tablespoons olive oil
- 1 onion, chopped
- 4 cloves garlic, minced
- 3 pinches dried rosemary
- Ground black pepper to taste
- 1 lemon, halved

Directions:

1. Preheat oven to 350 degrees F.

2. Place cod fillets on an 18x18-inch piece of aluminum foil; top with oil. Sprinkle onion, garlic, rosemary, and pepper over oil and cod. Squeeze juice from ½ lemon evenly on top.

3. Lift up bottom and top ends of the aluminum foil towards the center; fold together to 1 inch above the cod. Flatten short ends of the aluminum foil; fold over to within 1 inch of the sides of the cod. Place foil package on a baking sheet.

4. Bake in the preheated oven until haddock flakes easily with a fish, about 45 minutes. Let sit, about 5 minutes. Open ends of the packet carefully; squeeze juice from the remaining 1/2 lemon on top.

Nutrition: Calories 171, Total Fat 11.3g, Saturated Fat 1.6g, Cholesterol 95mg, Sodium 308mg, Total Carbohydrate 5g, Dietary Fiber 1.1g, Total Sugars 1.6g, Protein 14.3g, Calcium 31mg, Iron 1mg, Potassium 76mg, Potassium 67mg

48. Honey Fish

Preparation Time: 15 min

Cooking Time: 30 minutes

Servings: 4

Ingredients:

- 3/4 cup olive oil, divided
- 1 1/2 pounds haddock, patted dry
- 1/2 cup honey
- 1 teaspoon dried basil

Directions:

1. Preheat oven to 400 degrees F.
2. Place 1/2 cup oil in a shallow microwave-safe bowl. Heat in the microwave until hot, about 30 seconds. Dip haddock in cracker mixture until coated on both sides. Transfer to a shallow baking dish.
3. Bake haddock in the preheated oven until flesh flakes easily with a fork, about 25 minutes.
4. Place remaining 1/4 cup oil in a small microwave-safe bowl. Heat in the microwave until hot, about 15 seconds. Stir in honey and basil until blended.
5. Remove haddock from the oven; drizzle honey oil on top.
6. Continue baking until top is browned, about 5 minutes more.

Nutrition: Calories 347, Total Fat 25.9g, Saturated Fat 3.6g, Cholesterol 16mg, Sodium 46mg, Total Carbohydrate 27.5g, Dietary Fiber 0.2g, Total Sugars 24.5g, Protein 5.6g, Calcium 11mg, Iron 4mg, Potassium 108mg, Potassium 97mg

POULTRY RECIPES

49. Basic "Rotisserie" Chicken

Preparation Time: 15 minutes

Cooking Time: 6 to 8 hours

Servings: 6

Ingredients:

- 1 teaspoon garlic powder
- 1 teaspoon chili powder
- 1 teaspoon paprika
- 1 teaspoon dried thyme leaves
- 1 teaspoon sea salt
- Pinch cayenne pepper
- Freshly ground black pepper
- 1 (4-5 lb.) whole chicken, neck and giblets removed
- ½ medium onion, sliced

Directions:

1. In a small bowl, stir together the garlic powder, chili powder, paprika, thyme, salt, and cayenne. Season with black pepper, and stir again to combine. Rub the spice mix all over the exterior of the chicken.
2. Place the chicken in the cooker with the sliced onion sprinkled around it.
3. Cover the cooker and set to low. Cook for at least 6 to 8 hours, or until the internal temperature reaches

165ºF on a meat thermometer and the juices run clear, and serve.

Nutrition: Calories: 862 Total Fat: 59g Total Carbs: 7g Sugar: 6g Fiber: 0g Protein: 86g Sodium: 1,200mg

50. Tangy Barbecue Chicken

Preparation Time: 15 minutes

Cooking Time: 3-4 hours

Servings: 4

Ingredients:

- 4- 5 (2 lb.)boneless, skinless chicken breasts
- 2 cups Tangy Barbecue Sauce with Apple Cider Vinegar

Directions:

1. In your slow cooker, combine the chicken and barbecue sauce. Stir until the chicken breasts are well coated in the sauce.
2. Cover the cooker and set to high. Cook for 3 to 4 hours, or until the internal temperature of the chicken reaches 165°F on a meat thermometer and the juices run clear.
3. Shred the chicken with a fork, mix it into the sauce, and serve.

Nutrition: Calories: 412 Total Fat: 13g Total Carbs: 22g Sugar: 19g Fiber: 0g Protein: 51g Sodium: 766mg

51. <u>Salsa Verde Chicken</u>

Preparation Time: 15 minutes

Cooking Time: 6 to 8 hours

Servings: 4

Ingredients:

- 4 to 5 boneless, skinless chicken breasts (about 2 pounds)
- 2 cups green salsa
- 1 cup chicken broth
- 2 tablespoons freshly squeezed lime juice
- 1 teaspoon sea salt
- 1 teaspoon chili powder

Directions:

1. In your slow cooker, combine the chicken, salsa, broth, lime juice, salt, and chili powder. Stir to combine.
2. Cover the cooker and set to low. Cook for at approximately 6 to 8 hours, or until the internal temperature of the chicken reaches 165°F on a meat thermometer and the juices run clear.
3. Shred the chicken with a fork, mix it into the sauce, and serve.

Nutrition: Calories: 318 Total Fat: 8g Total Carbs: 6g Sugar: 2g Fiber: 1g Protein: 52g Sodium: 1,510mg

MEAT RECIPES

52. Spicy Lamb Curry

Preparation Time: 15 minutes

Cooking Time: 2 hours 15 minutes

Servings: 6-8

Ingredients:

- 4 teaspoons ground coriander
- 4 teaspoons ground coriander
- 4 teaspoons ground cumin
- ¾ teaspoon ground ginger
- 2 teaspoons ground cinnamon
- ½ teaspoon ground cloves
- ½ teaspoon ground cardamom
- 2 tablespoons sweet paprika
- ½ tablespoon cayenne pepper
- 2 teaspoons chili powder
- 2 teaspoons salt
- 1 tablespoon coconut oil
- 2 pounds boneless lamb, trimmed and cubed into 1-inch size
- Salt
- ground black pepper
- 2 cups onions, chopped
- 1¼ cups water
- 1 cup of coconut almond milk

Directions:

1. For spice mixture in a bowl, mix all spices. Keep aside. Season the lamb with salt and black pepper.
2. Warm oil on medium-high heat in a large Dutch oven. Add lamb and stir fry for around 5 minutes. Add onion and cook approximately 4-5 minutes.
3. Stir in the spice mixture and cook approximately 1 minute. Add water and coconut almond milk and provide some boil on high heat.
4. Adjust the heat to low and simmer, covered for approximately 1-120 minutes or until the lamb's desired doneness. Uncover and simmer for about 3-4 minutes. Serve hot.

Nutrition: Calories: 466 Fat: 10g Carbohydrates: 23g Protein: 36g Potassium 599 mg Sodium 203 mg Phosphorus 0mg

53. Roast Beef

Preparation Time: 25 minutes

Cooking Time: 55 minutes

Servings: 3

Ingredients:

- Quality rump or sirloin tip roast
- Pepper & herbs

Directions:

1. Place in a roasting pan on a shallow rack. Season with pepper and herbs. Insert meat thermometer in the center or thickest part of the roast.
2. Roast to the desired degree of doneness. After removing from over for about 15 minutes, let it chill. In the end, the roast should be moister than well done.

Nutrition: Calories 158 Protein 24 g Fat 6 g Carbs 0 g Phosphorus 206 mg Potassium 328 mg Sodium 55 mg

BROTHS, CONDIMENT AND SEASONING

54. Poultry Seasoning

Preparation Time: 15 minutes

Cooking Time: 0 minutes

Servings: ½ cup

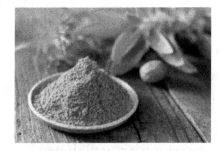

Ingredients:

- 2 tablespoons ground thyme
- 2 tablespoons ground marjoram
- 1 tablespoon ground sage
- 1 tablespoon ground celery seed
- 1 teaspoon ground rosemary
- 1 teaspoon freshly ground black pepper

Directions:

1. Mix the thyme, marjoram, sage, celery seed, rosemary, and pepper in a small bowl. Store for up to 6 months.

Nutrition: Calories: 3 Fat: 0g Carbohydrates: 0g Phosphorus: 3mg Potassium: 10mg Sodium: 1mg Protein: 0g

55. Berbere Spice Mix

Preparation Time: 15 minutes

Cooking Time: 4 minutes

Servings: ½ cup

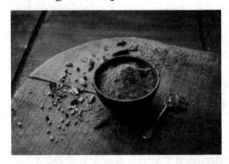

Ingredients:

- 1 tablespoon coriander seeds
- 1 teaspoon cumin seeds
- 1 teaspoon fenugreek seeds
- ¼ teaspoon black peppercorns
- ¼ teaspoon whole allspice berries
- 4 whole cloves
- 4 dried chilis, stemmed and seeded
- ¼ cup dried onion flakes
- 2 tablespoons ground cardamom
- 1 tablespoon sweet paprika
- 1 teaspoon ground ginger
- ½ teaspoon ground nutmeg
- ½ teaspoon ground cinnamon

Directions:

1. Put the coriander, cumin, fenugreek, peppercorns, allspice, and cloves in a small skillet over medium heat. Lightly toast the spices, swirling the skillet frequently, for about 4 minutes or until the spices are fragrant.

2. Remove the skillet, then let the spices cool for about 10 minutes. Transfer the toasted spices to a blender with the chilis and onion, and grind until the mixture is finely ground.

3. Transfer the ground spice mixture to a small bowl and stir together the cardamom, paprika, ginger, nutmeg, and cinnamon until thoroughly combined. Store the spice mixture in a small container with a lid for up to 6 months.

Nutrition: Calories: 8 Fat: 0gCarbohydrates: 2g Phosphorus: 7mg Potassium: 37mg Sodium: 14mg Protein: 0g

DRINKS AND SMOOTHIES

56. Distinctive Pineapple Smoothie

Preparation Time: 5 minutes

Cooking Time: 0 minutes

Servings: 2

Ingredients:

- ¼ cup crushed ice cubes
- 2 scoops vanilla whey protein powder
- 1 cup water
- 1½ cups pineapple

Directions:

1. In a high-speed blender, add all ingredients and pulse till smooth.

2. Transfer into 2 serving glass and serve immediately.

Nutrition: Calories 117 Fat 2.1g Carbs 18.2g Protein 22.7g Potassium (K) 296mg Sodium (Na) 81mg Phosphorous 28 mg

57. Strengthening Smoothie Bowl

Preparation Time: 5 minutes

Cooking Time: 4 minutes

Servings: 2

Ingredients:

- ¼ cup fresh blueberries
- ¼ cup fat-free plain Greek yogurt
- 1/3 cup unsweetened almond milk
- 2 tbsp. of whey protein powder
- 2 cups frozen blueberries

Directions:

1. In a blender, add blueberries and pulse for about 1 minute.
2. Add almond milk, yogurt and protein powder and pulse till desired consistency.
3. Transfer the mixture into 2 bowls evenly.
4. Serve with the topping of fresh blueberries.

Nutrition: Calories 176 Fat 2.1g Carbs 27g Protein 15.1g Potassium (K) 242mg Sodium (Na) 72mg Phosphorous 555.3 mg

DESSERT

58. Gingerbread loaf

Preparation time: 20 minutes

Cooking time: 1 hour

Servings: 16

Ingredients:

- Unsalted butter, for greasing the baking dish
- 3 cups all-purpose flour
- ½ teaspoon ener-g baking soda substitute
- 2 teaspoons ground cinnamon
- 1 teaspoon ground allspice
- ¾ cup granulated sugar
- 1¼ cups plain rice almond milk
- 1 large egg
- ¼ cup olive oil
- 2 tablespoons molasses
- 2 teaspoons grated fresh ginger
- Powdered sugar, for dusting

Directions:

1. Preheat the oven to 350°f.

2. Lightly grease a 9-by-13-inch baking dish with butter; set aside.

3. In a large bowl, sift together the flour, baking soda substitute, cinnamon, and allspice.

4. Stir the sugar into the flour mixture.

5. In medium bowl, whisk together the almond milk, egg, olive oil, molasses, and ginger until well blended.

6. Make a well in the center of the flour mixture and pour in the wet ingredients.

7. Mix until just combined, taking care not to overmix.

8. Pour the batter into the baking dish and bake for about 1 hour or until a wooden pick inserted in the middle comes out clean.

9. Serve warm with a dusting of powdered sugar.

Nutrition: calories: 232; fat: 5g; carbohydrates: 42g; phosphorus: 54mg; potassium: 104mg; sodium: 18mg; protein: 4g

59. Elegant lavender cookies

Preparation Time: 10 minutes

Cooking time: 15 minutes

Servings: makes 24 cookies

Ingredients:

- 5 dried organic lavender flowers, the entire top of the flower
- ½ cup granulated sugar
- 1 cup unsalted butter, at room temperature
- 2 cups all-purpose flour
- 1 cup rice flour

Directions:

1. Strip the tiny lavender flowers off the main stem carefully and place the flowers and granulated sugar into a food processor or blender. Pulse until the mixture is finely chopped.

2. In a medium bowl, cream together the butter and lavender sugar until it is very fluffy.

3. Mix the flours into the creamed mixture until the mixture resembles fine crumbs.

4. Gather the dough together into a ball and then roll it into a long log.

5. Wrap the cookie dough in plastic and refrigerate it for about 1 hour or until firm.

6. Preheat the oven to 375°f.

7. Slice the chilled dough into ¼-inch rounds and refrigerate it for 1 hour or until firm.

8. Bake the cookies for 15 to 18 minutes or until they are a very pale, golden brown.

9. Let the cookies cool.

10. Store the cookies at room temperature in a sealed container for up to 1 week.

Nutrition: calories: 153; fat: 9g; carbohydrates: 17g; phosphorus: 18mg; potassium: 17mg; sodium: 0mg; protein: 1g

60. Carob angel food cake

Preparation Time: 30 minutes

Cooking time: 30 minutes

Servings: 16

Ingredients:

- ¾ cup all-purpose flour
- ¼ cup carob flour
- 1½ cups sugar, divided
- 12 large egg whites, at room temperature
- 1½ teaspoons cream of tartar
- 2 teaspoons vanilla

Directions:

1. Preheat the oven to 375°f.
2. In a medium bowl, sift together the all-purpose flour, carob flour, and ¾ cup of the sugar; set aside.
3. Beat the egg whites and cream of tartar with a hand mixer for about 5 minutes or until soft peaks form.
4. Add the remaining ¾ cup sugar by the tablespoon to the egg whites until all the sugar is used up and stiff peaks form.
5. Fold in the flour mixture and vanilla.
6. Spoon the batter into an angel food cake pan.
7. Run a knife through the batter to remove any air pockets.

8. Bake the cake for about 30 minutes or until the top springs back when pressed lightly.

9. Invert the pan onto a wire rack to cool.

10. Run a knife around the rim of the cake pan and remove the cake from the pan.

Nutrition: calories: 113; fat: 0g; carbohydrates: 25g; phosphorus: 11mg; potassium: 108mg; sodium: 42mg; protein: 3g

CPSIA information can be obtained
at www.ICGtesting.com
Printed in the USA
LVHW011211090621
689781LV00002B/188